Healthy Nutrition For Life!

A Nutrition Guide to Weight Loss for You and Your Family

Author: Chris Alexander

Edited By:

Barry Kephart & Aaron
Christiano

Disclaimer

The advice contained herein is mentioned in a neutral manner. It is understood that the reader claims responsibility for their own actions and interpretations of the advice mentioned herein.

The author does not claim nor was any guarantee made regarding any success through this book. Therefore they cannot be held responsible should any losses, risks, liability or damages that might be linked, directly or indirectly, with the information contained within this book should occur.

Contents

What Being Healthy Means

"Either we suffer in health, we suffer in soul or we get fat."

When it comes to your health, there can be a broad definition to the term. Many people understand you need to have the best possible life in order to have a good time. There are a few things that can make a huge impact on you other than focusing on those aspects that allow you to have a healthier, happier life.

You also need to be healthy in more ways than one. When it comes down to it, many people assume they are healthy without actually knowing what true health is like. Moreover, for many people, being healthy is completely different.

Being healthy relies on a mix of mental and physical elements that enable the body to be the best it can be. Being healthy also depends upon a person being well mentally, physically and spiritually capable of having a good mindset. However, many people believe being healthy means having no diseases in the body.

Physical fitness can have a huge impact on your health but it is not the only thing. Being fit makes it easier for you to feel well, to feel good about your body. On the other hand, if your mind is deteriorating, then you will be unable to function properly. Proper mind, body and physical fitness need to be aligned right in order to allow a person to feel healthy about themselves.

In life, everyone has their own goals and what they want and do not want. Luckily for you, what you have to realize is the fact that there can be loads of ways you look after yourself. You can't really live your life if you aren't healthy.

When it comes down to it, being healthy is a state of mind. When you have your health, you can work towards having better goals in life.

Health and Short-Term and Long-Term Goals in Lives

Good health is always coupled with short-term and long-term goals in your lives. The long-term goals one has are the main reason for why good health is a necessity.

Live Longer

For many people, it is an unquestioned fact that they will be able to live a better life. When you have a healthy life, you can work on making things better for yourself. On the other hand, when you take the time to look good, you feel good as well.

This is why you can invest in your health and have a better time as well. In a report published by the Library of Science Medicine and Public, you can find that people who exercise well, drink alcohol in moderation and have a nutritious diet and avoid smoking, they actually end up with better life expectancy.

When you live to be a 100, you will be oblivious to the fact that life can get frustrating. On the other hand, all that is not going to matter if you haven't even made things worthwhile or enjoyed the fruits of your labor.

When you look after yourself well, you will be able to enjoy life to the fullest. A strong and healthy body will allow you to go after your goals.

More Energy

While exercise can make you feel fatigued, this fatigue is actually good for you. As your muscles repair themselves and recover, they become stronger and more robust. There are certain ways this might seem counterintuitive to you but you have to realize that these things can actually work to your benefit.

Whether you take a quick walk around the block or do yoga, embark on a hike in solitude. You will feel like the exercise is working out for you. Why? Mainly because you get to release some feel good endorphins that will make you feel better and improve your energy levels as well.

Avoid Disease or Illness

Apart from making you look good, you will realize your routine of eating right, being healthy and having a diet that releases you from toxins or diseases is free from infections.

A good lifestyle helps you get rid of hypertension and high blood pressure. This also reduces the chances of developing high cholesterol, eliminate diabetes and keep your heart in shape as well.

Keep Your Medical Costs Down

A medical study also showcased that people who have better weight can actually lower the chances of having lower medical costs. When you are healthy, you tend to have a healthier lifestyle that keeps your body working better than expected. On that note try your hardest to eat and live better as well.

Kids and Grandkids

Many people want to be there to see the various milestones that come throughout life. These milestones are apparent in the graduations, weddings, proms and birthdays of their children and grandchildren.

When you look after yourself, you make it possible for your body, mind, and health to age well and give you a better outlook on things.

Empowerment and Confidence

When you keep your body healthy, you will be able to feel good about yourself. This will also give you the confidence and empowerment you needed in order to lead a better life.

Look Better

When you look better, you feel better too. However, looking good is not only limited to how well you look in a layer of clothes. Many have goals to be able to look better with a beach body!

However, when you are truly in shape, you will be able to look good in anything without feeling like you look bad. With the help of these things, you can ensure you feel good about yourself. You appearance will also be affected by it, allowing you to have better hair, teeth and skin overall.

Better Mental Health

At Duke University, a study was done in order to find out just exactly where and when someone is. With the help of these things, it was found that among the students, over 60% were able to successfully overcome their depression by using anti-depressants.

Exercise also makes it possible to have better mental health and one can truly benefit from it without worrying about any negative side effects.

Why We Eat

Eating is a basic human urge that makes it possible for us to have a functional body. This does not mean we need to feed the body just any old meal. We have to take care what we feed ourselves.

The body needs fuel to continue functioning properly and if you aren't eating right, then your body won't be functioning right. With proper nutrition, you feed your body and keep it working effectively in order to ensure all your bodily functions are going right.

Difference between Hunger, Satiation and Overeating

Food is eaten in order to satisfy the body and the hunger one feels. This is in order to provide the body with the essential nutrients, energy and other substances the body needs to grow and maintain a healthy life.

When we feel hungry, it is our stomach's way of letting us know we need to re-fuel with something tasty and good for ourselves. . Once it runs out of fuel, you will start to feel hungry once again.

Satiation depends on the sensation of fullness the stomach experiences when the body has had enough food. This process depends on the receptors of the body that allows the stomach to know when it is full or when it is empty. This is also an important "health related" fact. Eat until you are satisfied. There is no need to stuff yourself at every meal and in fact eating until you are uncomfortably full at every meal is very unhealthy.

How Much Should We Eat?

Men and women have different needs. These nutritional needs vary from person to person. Caloric intake(the amount of calories of food you eat each day) will fluctuate with yours goals, your lifestyle(how active you are) and even change from day to day. By this we mean that if you are very active on Saturday playing Beach Volley ball all day, you will be a bit hungrier because you have burned so many calories that day. On Sunday you may not be as active and won't have burned so much energy.

Adjusting your eating habits based on your day is a very good way help lose weight. Just remember, you won't need all that extra food on rest days or easy days compared to your harder or more active days.

If you want to lose weight or determine a personal healthy weight for your lifestyle. Take any type of weight loss plans very seriously and step by step. There are no shortcuts to weight loss and you should never try to starve yourself with a huge "caloric deficit" to try and lose weight.

The main point to focus on is you have to realize how much you should eat and this can be based largely on your body weight and a wide range of factors, such as your size and how active you are physically.

An Eating Routine

An eating routine needs to be established in order to have the best things possible out of life. There are few things that can affect your weight but your eating routine is definitely among the things that matter.

Adjusting your meals to match your level of activity, while ensuring you are getting all essential nutrients and vitamins and minerals, is the most important and hardest goal. It takes time to dial in where you need to be to both be at a comfortable weight(or lose some of it) and to be strong and healthy.

Balanced Diet

When eating or drinking, you will often have to pay attention to the food you consume throughout the day. It's not just one meal, drink or snack but your entire meal plan that needs to be watched and adjusted when and if needed.

Good, healthy food is not fast food or junk food but food that will fill the basic health needs that the body has. Meals made to create a balanced diet are generally the best idea. On the other hand, there are many things that do not allow for a person to eat the proper food they need. Such as allergies for a particular food or not really liking a food based on taste or texture.

Junk food, fast food, pre-cooked easy meals and other items are more affordable but they are packed with calories, fatty acids, that do not complete a balanced diet. While it is not terrible to eat an unhealthy meal irregularly, it is not recommended, for a full and healthy lifestyle, to eat "junk food" every day.

An Active Metabolism

Another thing that actively affects the amount of food you consume is the metabolism you have. People with higher metabolisms can generally eat more without worrying about their calorie intake as much. However, the faster metabolism must still be fed by foods that are healthy and fit into that well balanced diet.

In fact, one might have to eat several small meals throughout the day in order to avoid their stomach growling all the time. The more active your metabolism is, the better your body will digest everything and make it possible for you to maintain the proper body weight.

What We Eat

Eating well is never the proper solution if you are not eating right. Any meal that you consume should have the following components:

Macronutrients

Like anything in life, food consists of various nutrients and macronutrients that are its building blocks. In short, they are the very essence of the energy your body needs. All food you consume is broken down into these the following macronutrients that your body needs.

Carbohydrates (4 Calories per Gram)

Carbohydrates are the bad guys in the diet industry at the moment. Many people are also under the impression that all carbs are bad for the body. Unfortunately, such huge generalization of carbohydrates can worsen things since you might be tempted to cut them out. Carbs can be of two kinds and you need a healthy amount of both in your diet.

Simple Carbs

Simple carbs are exactly that. They are simple and are easily absorbed into the blood stream of the body. They are largely found in organic fruits, vegetables and grass grown meat products.

Complex Carbs

These are different and have a molecular composition that makes it difficult for them to be absorbed into the blood stream. Complex carbs are also a necessary part of nutrition. In other words though, complex carbs consist of fibers and starches in the body while simple carbs.

Protein (4 Calories per Gram)

Proteins are an essential part of the building blocks in your body and require some time and effort on your part. Necessary for the body in order to keep, maintain, build and enable healthy protein functions in the body, a good amount of protein is necessary.

Fats (9 Calories per Gram)

Once again, much like carbohydrates, the fats in the body are accused of being unhealthy for the body. Once again though, you need to know your fats. Certain fats are healthy and necessary for the body while certain fats are not.

Bad Fats

Among the bad fats, you have to pay attention to the fact that certain fats are harmful for the body. They play a major role in helping the body develop, repair and produce healthy elevated fats.

Saturated Fats

Saturated fats are the unhealthy type of fats that is commonly found from natural animal and plant based sources. These fats can be responsible for promoting and increasing the risk of suffering from high cholesterol and various heart diseases. Popular sources of saturated fats are butter, cheese, palm and coconut oil and chicken with skin.

Trans Fats

These fats are a huge no-no and should be generally avoided. These are the ones that are generally found in junk food and frozen food items. Trans fats and saturated fats are usually solid at room temperature.

Good Fats

While many people tend to find it easier to avoid all fats and simply focus on eating a diet that has no fats, your body still needs them. Therefore, the best option is to consider opting for good fats.

Monounsaturated Fats

Mono unsaturated fats are found from plant sources other than coconut and palm oil. Oils derived from seeds and nuts all come under mono unsaturated fats. These are easier to digest and your body can easily digest them as well.

Polyunsaturated Fats

Similar to monounsaturated fats, these are beneficial for the body but are also meant to be eaten in moderation. These fats can affect your health in more ways than one.

Polyunsaturated fats can also help cut down on the buildup of unhealthy fats and cholesterol in the bloodstream and make it possible to have a healthier circulatory system.

Focusing on Quality Carbs, Proteins and Fats

At the end of the day, your diet should be focused around giving and getting quality nutrients to your body. With the help of this, you should be able to have a better life and focus on giving yourself a healthier alternative.

Luckily, you can also make it easier to have a better time. When you give, you get a lot of things back as well and when you invest the right proteins, carbs and fats in your body, you will be able to have a better body because of it.

What Is a Fad Diet?

When you are looking to incorporate a healthy diet, do your best to stay away from fad diets. Fad diets are basically the latest, best weight loss in the shortest number of days possible. A lot of people get duped into trying out these fad diets, mainly because they happen to promise such major results.

However, one untold and often overlooked fact remains true that there are certain fads that are not only ineffective but they are also harmful to the body. Each year, new fad diets are being introduced into the market and out of the given, there are very few that actually produce tangible results. The following are some of the most popular fad diets in the market:

High Carb

These diets focus on incorporating a high amount of carbs in the body. Since carbs are used to make energy in the body, with the help of this diet, one is promised optimum results, particularly if they are working out a lot.

Low Carb

These are complete opposites of high carb diets. Low carb diets focus on only giving the body a minimum amount of carbs. With this diet, they successfully limit the intake of the diet and make it possible to only give the body as much carbs as it needs to keep it fueled. The aim lies in only giving the body as many carbs as it needs instead of overfeeding it.

No Carb

In this fad diet, all carbs are deemed bad for the body and one sustains the body on a diet without any carbs at all. In this diet though, the damage one can do to their body is higher since a person can sustain more damage to themselves because the body does need a certain amount of carbs in order to function properly.

High Protein

Since proteins are also good for the body, high protein diets are hugely touted in fad diets as the next best thing. This is owing to the fact that these fad diets are meant for people who are looking to either bulk up faster or get leaner. Results can vary greatly, particularly if they are not coupled with the right exercises.

Only Protein

Again a fad diet that helps in focusing on getting leaner or to bulk up easily, it is necessary to have a good amount of protein. However, this fad diet revolves around only incorporating food items that have a good amount of protein in their diet.

Calorie Counting

Some diets simply focus on how many calories a meal has. This allows one to meet the total calorie count of the diet without wondering about the carbs, proteins and fats in the meal. While in many cases, this can be the best way possible to keep a check on your dietary and caloric needs.

Fad Diets - The Good, the Bad and the Ugly

When it comes down to it, fad diets look very good and flashy. While the ones mentioned above are the most common, it is possible to find different variations of these diets in the market.

Now fad diets are very hard to resist because their main marketing gimmick is the promise of fast and effective results. Do your best to make an educated guess regarding these diets and take the following things into account:

Very Extreme Eating or Lifestyle Change

The main thing to consider here is that you will need to make certain changes, in your lifestyle in order to have a radical change in your lifestyle. Your body is not going to be capable of losing weight in one day and if you put it through that unnecessary amount of strain, you will end up making things worse.

Moderation is Key

If fad diets are taken in moderation, you can get to see the promised results efficiently. With fad diets, you might end up hurting your body in order to get the results you are after. Luckily, with the help of fad diets, in moderation, you will be able to give your body time to change accordingly.

The Cost of "Their" Food

With fad diets, one of the main reasons why they fail is owing to the fact that you need to buy certain supplements and vitamins that are specific for their diet only. Many diets are centered on the fact that they have some kind of super food that can give your body the results it needs.

Costly and expensive, various fad diets make sure to emphasis the fact that one cannot get the results they are looking for if they have are not buying the supplements, food recommendations or other variations that are provided with the diet.

Temporary Weight loss

The results one gains from these diets are often temporary that go away once you switch back to your normal diet and your normal regime.

A person can look for various ways to get their hands on these diets and the results they give can make one overlook the fact that the results these crash diets promise will not last if continuous effort is not put in to keep it up as well. In this case, the results will definitely be temporary at best.

One Shoe Doesn't Fit All

Fad diets may be marketed to the masses but they are at times not meant for everyone. While one particular diet may produce certain results with someone, another one may not produce any results at all.

Similarly, when considering a diet, it is best to pay attention to the dynamics of the diet first. This is necessary since the different metabolisms of the body will definitely come into play and a person will definitely find that the fad diet is not working properly for everyone.

Differentiating between the Good and the Bad

There are few things that effectively make it possible for these fad diets to actually be good for you but you need to be able to differentiate successfully between them. With fad diets, there happen to be too many bad diets that make it harder to pick a diet that works.

Certain diets can be good for you but then again, certain diets are also bad for you. What you have to do is realize that certain diets have specific benefits and it is possible to come across fad diets that do produce tangible results.

Nutrition Myths

When focusing on having a healthy diet with nutrition, you need to focus on the fact that there may be some nutritional myths mixed in with the facts as well. While it may be tempting to give in and believe them, you have to realize that they should be believed with a grain of salt. The following are some of them:

Don't Eat Past 6:00 Pm

There really is no given time limit to when you should eat or not. However, what you eat should be taken into consideration. Eating meals that have carbs, healthy fats and proteins will make it possible for a person to have a healthy metabolism.

Eating foods that are high in fats, carbs and lards can increase the chances of more weight gain since the stomach has not had a chance to digest the food before.

Eating Fat Makes You Fat

Eating fat does not make you fat but you do have to realize that there are different variations of fat. These can be remotely hard if you don't pay attention to these factors but it is possible to make sure you only consume fat that is healthy for your body. By paying attention to the kind of fats you are consuming, you can make it easier to ensure that eating fat, does not, in fact, make you fat.

Coffee Is Bad

In this case, coffee can yield different results for people based on various different factors. For people who have certain medical conditions like cholesterol and diabetes, coffee can, indeed, be rather bad. On the other hand, for some people, the right blend of coffee can often be better for their heart.

However, once again, take the whole situation in consideration. If the scenario is centered around the fact that you skip meals and instead replace them with coffee, then you really should stop doing that. On the other hand, having it once in a while is still okay.

Starches Are Bad

Some starches are bad but once again, some are necessary for the body. Like fats and coffee, the main thing to consider is that practicing moderation is necessary. Saturating your body with unhealthy starches can be disastrous. Similarly, not having enough starch in the body is also troublesome since your body will require them.

Risks of Poor Nutrition

When a person is not fueling their body or giving it the proper nutrition it needs, you are not only putting it at risk but also increasing the chances of having your body suffer from a variety of ailments that can make it important to pay attention to your diet. Diabetes

Too much processed fat, starches and other poor nutrients can slowly push the blood sugar level of the body. Diabetes happens to be among the most common ailment among people who unintentionally tend to have a high level of sugar in their body.

It is also linked with having a diet that is high in fats, starches and lards. Diabetes is a condition where there is little control and proper treatment is not possible. One must do their best to control the situation with medication.

High Blood Pressure

Bad nutrition also fluctuates with the blood pressure of the body and often leads to a person developing hypertension. When this happens, it is possible for one to silently experience heart problems and suffer from undetected heart conditions that can be very hazardous for the body. Foods that are high in salt, sugar and diary are responsible for these.

Increased Chance of Cancer

Bad nutrition can also be responsible for provoking and creating different forms of cancer. This is owing to the fact that poor nutrition can aggravate the body and actually activate certain cancer cells in the body.

Furthermore, this gives rise to various different scenarios since it is possible for one to aggravate various cancer cells in their body. Foods that have refined nitrates, sugars and oils should be limited or avoided as much as possible.

High Cholesterol

Diets that have are high in fat are also responsible for increasing the cholesterol levels in the body. This in turn leads to clogging the arteries and increasing the chances of developing heart diseases.

Moreover, high cholesterol put the circulatory system under a lot of pressure. High cholesterol levels can also be linked to many silent heart attacks and other problems that plague the body from time to time.

Vitamin Deficiencies

Gout, scurvy and other skin and body conditions can easily affect a person when they have poor nutrition. This is owing to the fact that a person's diet is not providing them with the vital and essential nutrients they needed in order for them to function properly.

Over time, these deficiencies will start to manifest themselves in ways that make it harder for them to corrected or treated. A proper nutritional diet makes it easy for a person to not only look good but also have a happier, healthier life and to have the best possible way to meet their true potential in life.

With a diet that meets all the nutritional wants and needs of the body, you can ensure that the body stays healthy in order to accomplish all that the mind has in store for it. For this purpose, you will have to really focus on having a diet that meets all the proper nutritional needs of your body.

www.ingramcontent.com/pod-product-compliance
Lightning Source LLC
Chambersburg PA
CBHW070934290526
45795CB00003B/1013